Gray No More

The Ultimate Anti-Gray Hair

Nutrition and Wellness Guide

HR Research Alliance

This book features large print to accommodate readers with visual impairments, ensuring a comfortable and accessible reading experience for everyone.

Follow us on Amazon – HR Research Alliance – Search for more titles by HR Research Alliance wherever Books, Audiobooks, & eBooks are sold.

After reading, if you have a brief moment to leave a review that would be so much appreciated.

Table of Contents

Introduction

Aging is a natural part of life, a journey we all embark on from the moment we are born. As the years go by, our bodies undergo numerous changes, some more visible than others. One of the most noticeable signs of aging is the gradual graying of hair. For many, this transition can be a reminder of the passage of time, while for others, it's simply a natural shift that comes with maturity.

Hair, often seen as a symbol of youth and vitality, undergoes its own aging process. The color of our hair is determined by the pigment melanin, produced by specialized cells called melanocytes. As we age, the activity of these cells slows down, leading to a decrease in melanin production. This results in the emergence of grey or white hair. While genetics play a significant role in when and how quickly this process occurs, other factors like oxidative stress, nutritional deficiencies, and lifestyle choices can accelerate the graying process.

But what if we could influence this process? What if the foods we eat and the nutrients we consume could help us maintain our natural hair color for longer? This guide book explores that possibility.

Why Diet Matters

The saying "you are what you eat" holds more truth than we might realize, especially when it comes to our hair. Just as our diet affects our skin, weight, and overall health, it also plays a crucial role in the health of our hair, including its color. Nutrients like vitamins, minerals, and antioxidants are essential for maintaining the health and vitality of our hair follicles and the melanocytes responsible for hair pigmentation.

In recent years, there has been a growing interest in how diet can influence aging, not just in terms of lifespan but also in the quality of life. More people are seeking natural ways to slow down the visible signs of aging, and diet is emerging as a powerful tool in this endeavor. While hair dye offers a temporary solution to grey hair, a diet rich in the right nutrients may provide a more lasting and holistic approach.

This guide delves into the science behind hair pigmentation and the nutrients that support it. We'll explore how incorporating specific foods into your diet can help you maintain your natural hair color, reduce the appearance of grey hair, and improve the overall health of your hair.

Who This Book Is For

This book is for anyone who is interested in taking a proactive, natural approach to aging—specifically, those who want to maintain their hair's natural color for as long as possible. It's especially targeted at middle-aged and senior readers who are beginning to notice the first signs of grey hair or who have already experienced a significant change in their hair color.

Whether you're just starting to see a few grey strands or have been dealing with greying hair for years, this book offers valuable insights and practical tips on how to use diet and lifestyle changes to support your hair's health. You'll learn about the key nutrients your hair needs, the foods that provide them, and how to incorporate these into your daily meals.

This isn't just about preventing or reducing grey hair; it's about embracing a holistic approach to aging that nourishes your body from the inside out. By making mindful choices about what you eat, you can support not only your hair but also your overall well-being as you age.

Understanding Hair and Aging

The way our hair looks, feels, and even behaves can tell a lot about our overall health and well-being. To understand how we can influence our hair as we age, it's important first to grasp the basics of hair pigmentation and the various factors that contribute to the graying process.

The Science of Hair Pigmentation

Hair gets its color from a pigment called melanin, produced by specialized cells known as melanocytes. These melanocytes are located in the hair follicles, which are small cavities in the skin from which each strand of hair grows. Melanin is the same pigment responsible for the color of our skin and eyes, and it comes in two types: eumelanin and pheomelanin. Eumelanin is responsible for black and brown hair, while pheomelanin gives hair red and yellowish hues. The specific blend and concentration of these two types of melanin determine the color of an individual's hair.

As hair grows, melanocytes inject melanin into the keratin, the protein that makes up hair strands. This process gives each hair its natural color. However, as we age, the activity of melanocytes decreases. Over time, these cells produce less melanin, and eventually, they may stop producing it altogether. This gradual reduction in melanin is what causes hair to turn grey or white.

Why Hair Turns Grey

The graying of hair is a complex process influenced by a variety of factors, both internal and external. While genetics is the most significant determinant of when and how much our hair turns grey, other factors also play a crucial role.

1. Genetics: The timing of when your hair starts to grey is largely written in your DNA. If your parents and grandparents turned grey early, there's a good chance you will too. Genetic predisposition determines the lifespan of your melanocytes and how long they continue to produce melanin.

2. Oxidative Stress: One of the primary contributors to premature graying is oxidative stress. This occurs when there's an imbalance between free radicals (unstable molecules that can damage cells) and the body's ability to neutralize them with antioxidants. Over time, oxidative stress can damage melanocytes,

reducing their ability to produce melanin and accelerating the graying process.

3. Nutrient Deficiencies: Certain vitamins and minerals are essential for maintaining the health of melanocytes and promoting melanin production. Deficiencies in key nutrients, such as vitamin B12, folic acid, copper, and iron, can lead to premature graying. For example, vitamin B12 deficiency is commonly associated with early onset of grey hair, as this vitamin plays a critical role in the production and maintenance of healthy hair.

4. Hormonal Changes: As we age, our hormone levels fluctuate, which can affect melanin production. For instance, decreased levels of certain hormones like estrogen and

testosterone can influence the rate at which hair turns grey.

5. Environmental Factors: Exposure to environmental pollutants, toxins, and UV radiation can also contribute to the graying of hair by increasing oxidative stress on hair follicles.

Beyond the Greys

While grey hair is often the most visible sign of aging, it's not the only change our hair undergoes as we grow older. Aging can also affect hair strength, thickness, and shine. Hair may become thinner, more brittle, and lose its luster, making it more challenging to manage and style.

However, diet can play a significant role in not only influencing hair color but also in maintaining the overall health of your hair. Nutrients that support melanin production often overlap with those that strengthen hair and enhance its shine. For example, proteins and amino acids are crucial for both melanin production and the structural integrity of hair strands. Antioxidants, which combat oxidative stress, also help maintain the shine and thickness of hair.

By understanding the underlying mechanisms, we can take a proactive approach to slow down or even partially reverse some of these changes through targeted dietary and lifestyle choices. In the following chapters we will delve deeper into the specific nutrients and foods that can help maintain your natural hair color and improve the overall health of your hair as you age.

Nutrients that Support Hair Pigmentation

Healthy, vibrant hair is a reflection of overall well-being, and the nutrients we consume play a crucial role in maintaining its color, strength, and shine. In this chapter, we'll explore the key nutrients that support hair pigmentation, focusing on how they contribute to melanin production and overall hair health.

B Vitamins

B vitamins are vital for many bodily functions, including energy production, nerve function, and the maintenance of healthy skin and hair. When it comes to hair pigmentation, certain B vitamins stand out as particularly important:

1. Vitamin B12: Vitamin B12 is essential for the formation of red blood cells and the

maintenance of the nervous system, but it also plays a critical role in the health of hair follicles. A deficiency in B12 can lead to premature graying, as this vitamin is involved in the production of DNA, including the genetic material in hair cells that influence pigmentation. Ensuring adequate intake of B12 can help support the continued production of melanin, thus maintaining natural hair color.

2. Folic Acid (Vitamin B9): Folic acid is another B vitamin that is crucial for cell division and growth. It works closely with B12 to produce DNA and RNA, which are vital for the proper functioning of hair follicles. Folic acid also helps in the synthesis of methionine, an amino acid that plays a role in the production of melanin. A deficiency in folic acid can disrupt

these processes, potentially leading to premature graying.

3. Biotin (Vitamin B7): Often touted as a "hair vitamin," biotin supports the health of hair, skin, and nails. It is involved in the metabolism of fatty acids and amino acids, which are essential for hair growth and strength. While biotin doesn't directly influence hair color, it supports overall hair health, making it less prone to damage and breakage, which can contribute to a more vibrant appearance.

Copper and Iron

Copper and iron are two minerals that play a significant role in the production and maintenance of melanin, the pigment responsible for hair color.

1. Copper: Copper is a trace mineral that is crucial for the enzymatic process that converts tyrosine (an amino acid) into melanin. Without sufficient copper, this process is less efficient, leading to a reduction in melanin production and, consequently, the appearance of grey hair. Copper also supports the overall structure of hair, helping to maintain its strength and elasticity.

2. Iron: Iron is essential for the transportation of oxygen throughout the body, including to the hair follicles. Adequate oxygen levels are necessary for the health and function of melanocytes, the cells that produce melanin. Iron deficiency, which is common among women and older adults, can lead to hair thinning, dullness, and premature graying.

Ensuring a balanced intake of iron can help maintain healthy hair pigmentation.

Antioxidants

Oxidative stress is one of the leading causes of premature aging, including the graying of hair. Antioxidants are compounds that neutralize free radicals, thereby protecting cells from damage. Several antioxidants are particularly beneficial for hair health:

1. Vitamin C: Vitamin C is a powerful antioxidant that helps protect the hair follicles from oxidative damage. It also plays a crucial role in the production of collagen, a protein that supports the structure of hair and skin. By reducing oxidative stress, vitamin C can help slow down the graying process and maintain the natural color of your hair.

2. Vitamin E: Vitamin E is another potent antioxidant that protects cells from oxidative damage. It also improves blood circulation in the scalp, ensuring that hair follicles receive the nutrients they need to produce melanin. Regular intake of vitamin E can support healthy hair pigmentation and overall hair quality.

3. Selenium: Selenium is a trace mineral that works synergistically with other antioxidants to protect hair follicles from damage. It is also involved in the proper functioning of the thyroid gland, which regulates hair growth and pigmentation. Selenium deficiency can contribute to the premature graying of hair, making it important to include selenium-rich foods in your diet.

Omega-3 Fatty Acids

Omega-3 fatty acids are essential fats that the body cannot produce on its own, making it necessary to obtain them through diet. These healthy fats are known for their anti-inflammatory properties and their role in supporting overall health, including that of the scalp and hair.

Omega-3 fatty acids help keep the scalp hydrated and reduce inflammation, which can negatively impact hair health. A healthy scalp environment is crucial for the proper functioning of hair follicles, including the melanocytes responsible for melanin production. Additionally, omega-3s help nourish hair, making it more resilient and shiny, which can enhance the appearance of your natural hair color.

Protein and Amino Acids

Hair is primarily made up of a protein called keratin, and amino acids are the building blocks of proteins. Adequate protein intake is essential for healthy hair growth and pigmentation.

1. Tyrosine: Tyrosine is an amino acid that plays a direct role in the production of melanin. It is a precursor to both eumelanin and pheomelanin, the pigments that give hair its color. Consuming foods rich in tyrosine, such as meat, dairy products, and certain seeds, can support melanin production and help maintain your natural hair color.

2. Cysteine: Cysteine is another amino acid that is important for the production of keratin. It helps strengthen hair and protect it from damage, which can contribute to a healthier appearance overall. Cysteine also plays a role in the body's antioxidant defenses, further supporting the health of hair follicles.

In summary, maintaining your natural hair color and overall hair health as you age is closely tied to the nutrients you consume. By ensuring an adequate intake of B vitamins, copper, iron, antioxidants, omega-3 fatty acids, and protein, you can support melanin production, protect against oxidative stress, and promote healthy hair growth. The following chapters will guide you on how to incorporate these nutrients into your diet through delicious and practical food choices.

Anti-Grey Hair Superfoods

The foods we eat play a crucial role in nourishing our bodies from the inside out, and when it comes to maintaining healthy, vibrant hair, the right nutrients can make all the difference. In this chapter, we'll explore some of the most potent superfoods that support hair health and pigmentation. These foods are rich in the vitamins, minerals, and antioxidants necessary to keep your hair strong, shiny, and full of color.

Top 10 Superfoods for Hair Health

1. Leafy Greens (Spinach, Kale, Swiss Chard)

Leafy greens are nutritional powerhouses, packed with vitamins A, C, and folic acid, as well as iron. These nutrients are essential for promoting healthy hair growth and maintaining the hair's natural color. Spinach and kale are particularly rich in iron and vitamin C, which help keep hair follicles strong and prevent premature graying.

2. Nuts (Almonds, Walnuts, Brazil Nuts)

Nuts are excellent sources of biotin, vitamin E, and healthy fats, all of which support hair health. Walnuts, in particular, are rich in omega-3 fatty acids and copper, both of which play a crucial role in maintaining hair pigmentation. Brazil nuts are one of the best dietary sources of selenium, a mineral that helps protect hair from oxidative stress.

3. Seeds (Flaxseeds, Chia Seeds, Pumpkin Seeds)

Seeds are tiny nutritional powerhouses loaded with essential fatty acids, zinc, and antioxidants. Flaxseeds and chia seeds are rich in omega-3 fatty acids, which help keep the scalp hydrated and reduce inflammation. Pumpkin seeds are high in zinc, a mineral that supports healthy hair follicles and may help prevent hair thinning and graying.

4. Eggs

Eggs are one of the best sources of protein and biotin, two nutrients essential for strong, healthy hair. They also contain vitamin B12 and iron, both of which are important for maintaining hair color and preventing premature graying. The combination of these nutrients makes eggs a perfect food for those looking to support their hair health.

5. Seafood (Salmon, Sardines, Oysters)

Seafood is rich in omega-3 fatty acids, vitamin D, and zinc, all of which contribute to healthy hair. Salmon and sardines provide high levels of omega-3s, which help reduce scalp inflammation and support hair growth. Oysters are particularly high in zinc and iron, two minerals that play a key role in maintaining hair pigmentation and preventing hair loss.

6. Berries (Blueberries, Strawberries, Raspberries)

Berries are packed with antioxidants, particularly vitamin C, which helps protect hair follicles from oxidative stress and supports collagen production. Blueberries are especially rich in vitamin C and anthocyanins, which help maintain the health of blood vessels, ensuring that hair follicles receive adequate nutrients and oxygen.

7. Avocado

Avocado is a nutrient-dense fruit rich in healthy fats, vitamin E, and B vitamins. These nutrients help nourish the scalp, support hair growth, and maintain the hair's natural color. The healthy fats in avocado also help keep hair hydrated and reduce breakage.

8. Sweet Potatoes

Sweet potatoes are an excellent source of beta-carotene, which the body converts into vitamin A. Vitamin A is essential for the production of sebum, an oily substance that keeps the scalp moisturized and hair healthy. Adequate vitamin A intake can also help maintain the health and pigmentation of hair follicles.

9. Lentils

Lentils are a great plant-based source of protein, iron, zinc, and biotin. These nutrients support hair growth, strengthen hair follicles, and maintain the natural color of hair. Lentils are also rich in folic acid, which is important for red blood cell production and the delivery of oxygen to hair follicles.

10. Yogurt

Yogurt is rich in protein, vitamin B5 (pantothenic acid), and vitamin D, all of which support hair health. The probiotics in yogurt also help maintain a healthy scalp by balancing the scalp's microbiome, which can reduce dandruff and promote hair growth.

Incorporating These Foods into Your Diet

Incorporating these superfoods into your daily meals can be simple and delicious. Here are some practical tips to help you add these nutrient-rich foods to your diet:

1. Smoothies: Start your day with a nutrient-packed smoothie by blending spinach, berries, avocado, and a scoop of yogurt. Add a tablespoon of flaxseeds or chia seeds for an extra boost of omega-3 fatty acids.

2. Salads: Create a colorful salad with leafy greens like kale or spinach, topped with nuts (almonds or walnuts), seeds (pumpkin or sunflower), and a portion of grilled salmon or sardines. Drizzle with olive oil and a squeeze of lemon for a tasty, hair-healthy meal.

3. Breakfast Bowls: Enjoy a breakfast bowl with scrambled eggs, avocado slices, and a side of sweet potato hash. This combination provides a good mix of protein, healthy fats, and beta-carotene to support your hair.

4. Snacks: Keep a handful of nuts and seeds on hand for a quick and easy snack that supports hair health. You can also snack on yogurt with a sprinkle of berries for added antioxidants.

5. Lentil Stews and Soups: Incorporate lentils into your diet by preparing hearty stews and soups. Combine lentils with vegetables like sweet potatoes and leafy greens for a filling and nutritious meal.

Spotlight on Herbs and Spices

Herbs and spices are not only flavorful additions to your meals but also powerful allies in promoting hair health. Here are some herbs and spices known for their hair-nourishing properties:

1. Curry Leaves: Curry leaves are rich in antioxidants, beta-carotene, and amino acids that help strengthen hair follicles and promote hair growth. They are also believed to help retain natural hair color and delay the graying process. Incorporate curry leaves into your cooking by adding them to curries, soups, or chutneys.

2. Amla (Indian Gooseberry): Amla is a traditional remedy for hair health in Ayurvedic medicine. It is rich in vitamin C and antioxidants, which help protect hair from oxidative stress and promote healthy hair growth. Amla can be consumed as a powder,

juice, or oil, and can also be added to smoothies or teas.

3. Black Sesame Seeds: Black sesame seeds are believed to have anti-aging properties and are often used in traditional medicine to maintain hair color and prevent graying. They are rich in minerals like copper and zinc, which support melanin production. Sprinkle black sesame seeds on salads, yogurt, or stir-fries for a nutty flavor and added nutrients.

Incorporating these superfoods, herbs, and spices into your diet can provide the essential nutrients your hair needs to stay healthy, strong, and full of color. By making these foods a regular part of your meals, you can take a proactive approach to maintaining your hair's natural vitality and delaying the signs of aging.

Meal Plans for Maintaining Hair Color

A well-structured meal plan can make it easier to incorporate the essential nutrients that support hair health and pigmentation into your daily diet. In this chapter, we'll provide a 7-day anti-grey hair diet plan, along with specific ideas for breakfasts, lunches, dinners, snacks, and smoothies. These meals are designed to be both delicious and nutrient-dense, helping you to maintain your natural hair color and overall vitality.

7-Day Anti-Grey Hair Diet Plan

Day 1

- Breakfast: Spinach and mushroom omelet with a side of whole-grain toast

- Lunch: Quinoa salad with avocado, cherry tomatoes, walnuts, and grilled chicken

- Dinner: Baked salmon with roasted sweet potatoes and steamed broccoli

- Snack: A handful of almonds and a small bowl of blueberries

- Smoothie: Kale, banana, chia seeds, and almond milk smoothie

Day 2

- Breakfast: Greek yogurt with mixed berries, flaxseeds, and honey

- Lunch: Lentil soup with a mixed green salad topped with sunflower seeds and vinaigrette

- Dinner: Stir-fried tofu with black sesame seeds, bell peppers, and brown rice

- Snack: Sliced apple with almond butter

- Smoothie: Spinach, pineapple, and coconut water smoothie

Day 3

- Breakfast: Oatmeal with sliced bananas, walnuts, and a sprinkle of cinnamon

- Lunch: Turkey and avocado wrap with whole-grain tortilla and a side of carrot sticks

- Dinner: Grilled shrimp with quinoa, sautéed kale, and lemon-garlic dressing

- Snack: Pumpkin seeds and a small piece of dark chocolate

- Smoothie: Blueberries, Greek yogurt, and flaxseed smoothie

Day 4

- Breakfast: Scrambled eggs with sautéed spinach and cherry tomatoes

- Lunch: Chickpea and spinach curry with brown rice

- Dinner: Baked cod with roasted Brussels sprouts and sweet potato mash

- Snack: A small handful of Brazil nuts

- Smoothie: Mango, turmeric, and coconut milk smoothie

Day 5

- Breakfast: Chia pudding made with almond milk, topped with strawberries and black sesame seeds

- Lunch: Grilled chicken Caesar salad with kale and a sprinkle of parmesan

- Dinner: Beef and vegetable stir-fry with bell peppers, broccoli, and brown rice

- Snack: Celery sticks with hummus

- Smoothie: Mixed berry, spinach, and almond butter smoothie

Day 6

- Breakfast: Avocado toast with poached eggs and a side of fresh fruit

- Lunch: Lentil and sweet potato stew with a side of steamed green beans

- Dinner: Baked turkey breast with roasted carrots and quinoa

- Snack: A small bowl of mixed nuts (almonds, walnuts, Brazil nuts)

- Smoothie: Kiwi, spinach, and Greek yogurt smoothie

Day 7

- Breakfast: Smoothie bowl with spinach, banana, blueberries, and granola

- Lunch: Grilled salmon with a side of quinoa salad and steamed asparagus

- Dinner: Roast chicken with a side of roasted root vegetables and a mixed green salad

- Snack: Sliced cucumbers with tzatziki dip

- Smoothie: Papaya, flaxseed, and almond milk smoothie

Breakfasts: Healthy, Nutrient-Dense Breakfast Ideas

1. Spinach and Mushroom Omelet: Sauté spinach and mushrooms in butter or coconut oil, then add beaten eggs. Cook until the eggs are set, and serve with whole-grain toast. This breakfast provides a good mix of protein, iron, and B vitamins.

2. Greek Yogurt with Berries and Flaxseeds: Top a bowl of Greek yogurt with mixed berries, a tablespoon of flaxseeds, and a drizzle of honey. This meal is rich in antioxidants, omega-3 fatty acids, and probiotics.

3. Oatmeal with Walnuts and Cinnamon: Cook oats in water or almond milk and top with sliced bananas, chopped walnuts, and a sprinkle of cinnamon. This breakfast is high in

fiber, healthy fats, and essential minerals like iron and magnesium.

4. Chia Pudding: Mix chia seeds with almond milk and let it sit overnight. In the morning, top with sliced strawberries and black sesame seeds for a nutrient-rich start to your day.

5. Avocado Toast with Poached Eggs: Spread mashed avocado on whole-grain toast and top with a poached egg. This breakfast is rich in healthy fats, protein, and B vitamins.

Lunches: Midday Meals that Nourish Hair from Within

1. Quinoa Salad with Avocado and Walnuts: Combine cooked quinoa with diced avocado, cherry tomatoes, walnuts, and grilled chicken. Toss with olive oil and lemon juice for a balanced and filling meal.

2. Lentil Soup with Mixed Greens: Prepare a hearty lentil soup with carrots, celery, and tomatoes. Serve with a side of mixed greens topped with sunflower seeds and a light vinaigrette.

3. Turkey and Avocado Wrap: Fill a whole-grain tortilla with sliced turkey, avocado, spinach, and a drizzle of mustard. Serve with carrot sticks for a fiber-rich lunch.

4. Chickpea and Spinach Curry: Cook chickpeas and spinach in a flavorful curry sauce made with onions, garlic, tomatoes, and spices. Serve with brown rice for a protein-packed meal.

5. Grilled Chicken Caesar Salad: Toss chopped kale with grilled chicken, a sprinkle of parmesan, and a light Caesar dressing. Add a side of whole-grain bread for a satisfying lunch.

Dinners: Balanced Meals for Optimal Hair Health

1. Baked Salmon with Roasted Sweet Potatoes: Season salmon fillets with herbs and bake until cooked through. Serve with roasted sweet potatoes and steamed broccoli for a meal rich in omega-3 fatty acids, vitamins, and minerals.

2. Stir-Fried Tofu with Black Sesame Seeds: Stir-fry tofu with bell peppers, snap peas, and garlic. Sprinkle with black sesame seeds and serve with brown rice for a plant-based dinner full of nutrients.

3. Grilled Shrimp with Quinoa and Kale**: Grill shrimp with a lemon-garlic marinade and serve over a bed of quinoa and sautéed kale. This dish is high in protein, iron, and antioxidants.

4. Baked Cod with Brussels Sprouts and Sweet Potato Mash: Bake cod fillets and serve with roasted Brussels sprouts and mashed sweet potatoes. This meal provides a good balance of protein, healthy fats, and vitamins.

5. Beef and Vegetable Stir-Fry: Stir-fry lean beef strips with bell peppers, broccoli, and onions in a soy-ginger sauce. Serve over brown rice for a filling and nutrient-dense dinner.

Snacks and Smoothies: Nutritious Snack Ideas and Recipes

1. Almonds and Blueberries: A small handful of almonds paired with a bowl of blueberries provides a perfect mix of healthy fats, fiber, and antioxidants.

2. Sliced Apple with Almond Butter: Dip apple slices in almond butter for a snack that's rich in vitamins, fiber, and healthy fats.

3. Pumpkin Seeds and Dark Chocolate: Enjoy a small portion of roasted pumpkin seeds with a piece of dark chocolate for a treat that's high in zinc, magnesium, and antioxidants.

4. Celery Sticks with Hummus: Dip crunchy celery sticks in hummus for a snack that's low in calories but high in fiber and protein.

5. Yogurt with Mixed Nuts: Top a bowl of Greek yogurt with mixed nuts and a drizzle of honey for a snack that's rich in probiotics, protein, and healthy fats.

Smoothie Recipes

1. Kale and Banana Smoothie: Blend kale, banana, chia seeds, and almond milk for a smoothie that's packed with vitamins, minerals, and omega-3 fatty acids.

2. Spinach and Pineapple Smoothie: Mix spinach, pineapple, and coconut water for a refreshing and antioxidant-rich drink.

3. Blueberry and Flaxseed Smoothie: Combine blueberries, Greek yogurt, flaxseeds, and water for a smoothie that's full of fiber, antioxidants, and protein.

4. Mango and Turmeric Smoothie: Blend mango, turmeric, and coconut milk for an anti-inflammatory and vitamin-rich smoothie.

5. Papaya and Flaxseed Smoothie: Mix papaya, flaxseed, and almond milk for a smoothie that supports digestion and hair health with its rich content of vitamins and healthy fats.

This 7-day meal plan and the included recipe ideas offer a variety of delicious and nutrient-dense options to support your hair health. By regularly incorporating these types of meals into your diet, you can nourish your hair from within, helping to maintain its natural color and vibrancy as you age.

Lifestyle Factors Affecting Hair Health

While diet plays a crucial role in maintaining hair health and color, lifestyle factors also significantly impact the vitality of your hair. This chapter explores how stress, sleep, exercise, and environmental factors can affect your hair, providing practical tips to help you maintain strong, healthy, and naturally vibrant hair as you age.

Stress Management

Chronic stress is a well-known contributor to various health issues, including premature graying and hair loss. When you experience stress, your body produces higher levels of cortisol, a hormone that can disrupt the normal functioning of hair follicles. This disruption can lead to a condition known as telogen effluvium, where hair prematurely enters the shedding phase, and can also accelerate the graying process.

To combat the effects of stress on your hair, it's important to incorporate relaxation techniques into your daily routine. Here are some effective strategies for managing stress:

1. Meditation: Regular meditation helps calm the mind, reduce stress, and promote overall well-being. Even just 10-15 minutes of daily meditation can have a positive impact on your stress levels. Consider guided meditation apps or attending a meditation class to get started.

2. Yoga: Yoga combines physical movement with mindfulness, making it an excellent practice for reducing stress. Certain yoga poses, such as the forward bend (uttanasana) and the

child's pose (balasana), are particularly effective at promoting relaxation and reducing tension in the body.

3. Breathing Exercises: Simple breathing exercises, such as deep breathing or the 4-7-8 technique, can help lower stress levels and promote a sense of calm. Practice these exercises during moments of stress or as part of your daily routine to support overall mental and physical health.

4. Mindfulness: Practicing mindfulness involves staying present and fully engaging in the current moment. This can be as simple as paying attention to your breath, taking a walk in nature, or focusing on a specific task without distractions. Mindfulness helps reduce stress and promotes a sense of peace and clarity.

5. Physical Activity: Regular physical activity is a natural stress reliever. Whether it's walking, swimming, or dancing, find an activity you enjoy and make it a part of your daily routine. Exercise helps release endorphins, the body's natural mood elevators, and can significantly reduce stress levels.

Sleep and Hair Health

Adequate sleep is essential for overall health, including the health of your hair. During sleep, your body goes through repair and regeneration processes, including the repair of hair follicles. Lack of sleep can disrupt these processes, leading to weakened hair, increased hair shedding, and even premature graying.

To improve your sleep quality and support hair health, consider the following tips:

1. Establish a Sleep Routine: Going to bed and waking up at the same time each day helps regulate your body's internal clock, making it easier to fall asleep and wake up feeling refreshed. Aim for 7-9 hours of sleep each night.

2. Create a Relaxing Sleep Environment: Your bedroom should be a calm and comfortable space conducive to sleep. Keep the room cool, dark, and quiet, and invest in a comfortable mattress and pillows. Consider using blackout curtains, earplugs, or a white noise machine if necessary.

3. Limit Screen Time Before Bed: The blue light emitted by phones, tablets, and computers can interfere with your body's production of melatonin, a hormone that regulates sleep. Try

to avoid screens at least an hour before bedtime and instead engage in relaxing activities like reading or listening to soothing music.

4. Avoid Stimulants Before Bed: Caffeine, nicotine, and heavy meals can disrupt your sleep. Try to avoid these stimulants in the evening and opt for a light snack if you're hungry before bed.

5. Practice Relaxation Techniques: Engage in relaxation techniques, such as deep breathing, progressive muscle relaxation, or a warm bath before bed to help your body unwind and prepare for sleep.

Exercise and Circulation

Regular exercise is not only beneficial for your overall health but also plays a significant role in promoting healthy hair. Exercise improves blood circulation, ensuring that essential nutrients and oxygen are delivered to the hair follicles. This increased blood flow helps support hair growth, strengthens hair strands, and can even enhance the vibrancy of your natural hair color.

Here's how you can incorporate exercise into your routine to support hair health:

1. Cardiovascular Exercise: Activities like walking, jogging, swimming, or cycling get your heart pumping and improve circulation throughout your body, including your scalp. Aim for at least 150 minutes of moderate-intensity cardio each week.

2. Strength Training: Strength training exercises, such as weightlifting or bodyweight exercises, help improve overall muscle tone and

boost circulation. Incorporate strength training into your routine 2-3 times a week to build muscle and promote healthy hair.

3. Scalp Massage: A simple scalp massage can help stimulate blood flow to the hair follicles. Use your fingertips to gently massage your scalp in circular motions for 5-10 minutes daily. You can also use essential oils, such as rosemary or peppermint oil, to enhance the massage and promote hair growth.

4. Yoga and Stretching: In addition to reducing stress, yoga and stretching exercises help improve flexibility and circulation. Certain yoga poses, such as the downward-facing dog (adho mukha svanasana) and the headstand (sirsasana), can specifically target blood flow to the scalp.

5. Stay Active: Beyond structured exercise, find ways to stay active throughout the day. Take the stairs instead of the elevator, go for a walk during lunch breaks, or do light stretching while watching TV. Staying active keeps your blood circulating and supports overall health.

Environmental Factors

The environment around us can have a significant impact on hair health. Factors such as pollution, sun exposure, and chemical treatments can damage hair, leading to dryness, brittleness, and premature graying. Understanding these environmental factors and taking steps to protect your hair can help maintain its health and natural color.

1. Pollution: Air pollution can deposit harmful particles on your hair and scalp, leading to

oxidative stress and weakening hair strands. To protect your hair from pollution, consider wearing a hat or scarf when outdoors, especially in heavily polluted areas. Regularly washing your hair with a gentle, sulfate-free shampoo can also help remove pollutants and keep your scalp clean.

2. Sun Exposure: Prolonged exposure to the sun's ultraviolet (UV) rays can damage the hair's cuticle, leading to dryness, split ends, and color fading. Protect your hair from sun damage by wearing a wide-brimmed hat. Additionally, limit prolonged direct sun exposure during peak hours (10 a.m. to 4 p.m.).

3. Chemical Treatments: Hair treatments such as coloring, perming, and straightening often involve harsh chemicals that can weaken hair

strands and strip them of their natural color. If you choose to undergo chemical treatments, make sure to space them out and follow up with deep conditioning treatments to help restore moisture and strength to your hair.

4. Chlorine and Saltwater: Chlorine in swimming pools and saltwater from the ocean can both dry out hair and cause it to become brittle. Before swimming, wet your hair and apply a leave-in conditioner to create a protective barrier. After swimming, rinse your hair thoroughly with fresh water and follow up with a hydrating conditioner.

5. Proper Hair Care: Regular hair care routines, such as gentle washing, conditioning, and avoiding excessive heat styling, can help maintain the health and appearance of your

hair. Use products that are suited to your hair type and avoid over-washing, which can strip hair of its natural oils.

By understanding and addressing these lifestyle factors, you can take proactive steps to maintain your hair's health, strength, and color. Stress management, quality sleep, regular exercise, and environmental protection are all integral parts of a holistic approach to hair care, helping you to keep your hair looking vibrant and youthful as you age.

Myth-Busting: What Works and What Doesn't

When it comes to maintaining hair color and delaying the graying process, there is no shortage of myths and misconceptions. In this chapter, we'll take a closer look at some of the most common myths about grey hair, discuss the pros and cons of supplements versus whole foods, and explore natural alternatives to chemical hair dyes. By separating fact from fiction, you'll be better equipped to make informed decisions about your hair care.

Common Myths about Grey Hair

Grey hair is a natural part of aging, but it has also become the subject of many myths. Let's debunk some of the most popular ones:

1. Myth: Plucking Grey Hairs Makes Them Multiply

- Fact: One of the most widespread myths is that plucking a grey hair will cause multiple grey hairs to grow in its place. The truth is, each hair follicle can only produce one hair at a time. Plucking a grey hair won't lead to more grey hairs, but it can damage the hair follicle and potentially cause thinning or scarring over time. It's best to avoid plucking altogether.

2. Myth: Stress Alone Causes Grey Hair

- Fact: While stress is often blamed for turning hair grey, it's not the sole cause. Genetics play the most significant role in determining when and how much grey hair you'll have. However, chronic stress can accelerate the process by contributing to oxidative stress, which damages cells, including those responsible for hair pigmentation.

3. Myth: Cutting Your Hair Frequently Will Prevent Greying

- Fact: The idea that regular haircuts can prevent or slow down the graying process is simply a myth. Haircuts have no impact on the color of your hair since hair growth and pigmentation occur at the follicle level beneath the scalp. While regular trims can keep your hair looking healthy, they won't influence whether your hair turns grey.

4. Myth: Only Older People Get Grey Hair

- Fact: While it's true that grey hair becomes more common with age, young people can also experience premature greying. This can be due to genetics, certain health conditions, or deficiencies in specific nutrients like vitamin B12. Premature greying is often hereditary and not necessarily a sign of poor health.

5. Myth: Grey Hair is Coarser and More Resistant to Styling

   - Fact: Some people believe that grey hair is inherently coarser and harder to manage. In reality, the texture of grey hair can vary widely. For some, it may become slightly coarser due to changes in the hair follicle, but for others, it may remain similar to their original hair texture. Proper hair care can help manage any changes in texture.

Supplements vs. Whole Foods

In the quest to maintain hair color and health, many people turn to supplements. However, it's important to weigh the benefits and limitations of supplements compared to getting nutrients from whole foods.

1. Supplements: Pros and Cons

- Pros: Supplements can be a convenient way to ensure you're getting specific nutrients that may be lacking in your diet, such as biotin, zinc, or B vitamins. They're particularly useful for individuals with dietary restrictions or health conditions that affect nutrient absorption.

- Cons: Supplements are not a substitute for a balanced diet. Relying too heavily on supplements can lead to nutrient imbalances or even toxicity, especially if taken in excessive amounts. Additionally, the body often absorbs nutrients from whole foods more effectively than from supplements, which means you may not get the full benefit of the vitamins and minerals in pill form.

2. Whole Foods: The Optimal Choice

- Pros: Whole foods provide a wide array of nutrients in their natural forms, along with fiber, antioxidants, and other beneficial compounds that work synergistically to support overall health, including hair health. Foods like leafy greens, nuts, seeds, and fatty fish are rich in the vitamins and minerals that promote healthy hair pigmentation.

- Cons: It can be challenging to get all the necessary nutrients from diet alone, especially if you have specific health concerns or dietary preferences. However, with a well-planned diet, it's entirely possible to meet your nutritional needs without the need for supplements.

In summary, while supplements can be helpful in certain situations, focusing on a diet rich in whole, nutrient-dense foods is the best way to support your hair health naturally. If you do choose to take supplements, it's wise to consult with a healthcare provider to ensure you're taking the right ones in appropriate doses.

Hair Dye Alternatives

For those looking to cover grey hair or enhance their natural color without resorting to chemical dyes, there are several natural alternatives worth exploring. These options are often gentler on the hair and scalp and can offer a more natural-looking result.

1. Henna

   - Overview: Henna is a plant-based dye that has been used for centuries to color hair naturally. It imparts a reddish-brown hue and can be mixed with other natural ingredients like indigo to achieve different shades.

- Effectiveness: Henna is effective at covering grey hair and can add richness and depth to natural hair color. It's also known for conditioning the hair, leaving it softer and shinier. However, it's important to note that henna works best on hair that is not overly processed or damaged.

- Considerations: Henna can be messy to apply and requires a longer processing time compared to chemical dyes. The color result can be unpredictable, especially if applied to very light or grey hair. Additionally, once henna is applied, it's challenging to remove, and it can limit the effectiveness of chemical dyes used afterward.

2. Indigo

- Overview: Indigo is another plant-based dye that is often used in conjunction with henna to achieve darker shades, such as brown or black. When used alone, indigo imparts a bluish tint to the hair.

- Effectiveness: Indigo is highly effective at darkening hair and covering grey when used properly. It's typically applied after a henna treatment to achieve the desired shade.

- Considerations: Like henna, indigo can be challenging to apply and requires patience. The color can be long-lasting, but it may fade over time, especially with frequent washing. As with henna, indigo should be used with caution if you plan to use chemical dyes in the future.

3. Herbal Rinses

- Overview: Herbal rinses made from ingredients like sage, rosemary, chamomile, and black tea can gradually darken hair and enhance natural tones. These rinses are typically used as a final rinse after shampooing.

- Effectiveness: Herbal rinses provide subtle, natural color enhancement and are less likely to cover grey hair completely. They work best for maintaining and enhancing existing color rather than making dramatic changes.

- Considerations: The results from herbal rinses are gradual and may require multiple applications to see noticeable changes. The color effect is temporary and will wash out over time, requiring regular use to maintain the desired shade.

4. Amla (Indian Gooseberry)

- Overview: Amla is a popular Ayurvedic remedy known for its hair-strengthening and color-enhancing properties. It's often used in powdered form or as an oil to condition hair and enhance its natural color.

- Effectiveness: Amla can help darken grey hair over time and improve overall hair texture and shine. It's also rich in vitamin C and antioxidants, which support scalp health and hair growth.

- Considerations: Amla is more of a conditioning treatment than a dye, so its color effects are subtle. It's best used as part of a broader hair care routine to maintain hair health and prevent further graying.

Natural hair dye alternatives offer a gentler approach to coloring hair, but they come with their own set of challenges. If you're looking for a natural way to maintain or enhance your hair color, it's important to have realistic expectations and be prepared for a bit of trial and error. These alternatives may not provide the same immediate or uniform results as chemical dyes, but they offer a healthier option for those who prefer a more natural approach to hair care.

In this chapter, we've dispelled common myths about grey hair, discussed the pros and cons of supplements versus whole foods, and explored natural alternatives to chemical dyes. Armed with this knowledge, you can make informed decisions about how to care for your hair and maintain its health and natural color.

Beyond Diet: Holistic Hair Care Practices

While diet is a critical component of maintaining healthy hair and preventing premature graying, it's equally important to adopt a holistic approach to hair care. This chapter explores the importance of scalp care, selecting the right hair care products, protective hairstyles, and DIY hair masks that can nourish and protect your hair. These practices, combined with a nutrient-rich diet, will help you achieve and maintain vibrant, healthy hair.

Scalp Care

A healthy scalp is the foundation for healthy hair. Proper scalp care ensures that your hair follicles receive the nutrients they need to produce strong, healthy hair strands. Here are some tips for maintaining a healthy scalp:

1. Gentle Scalp Massage: Regular scalp massages stimulate blood circulation, which helps deliver nutrients and oxygen to the hair follicles. Use your fingertips to gently massage your scalp in circular motions for 5-10 minutes a few times a week. You can enhance the experience by using essential oils like rosemary or lavender, which are known for promoting hair growth.

2. Natural Scalp Treatments: Incorporating natural treatments into your scalp care routine can address issues like dryness, dandruff, and excess oil production. Consider these natural options:

- Aloe Vera: Aloe vera has soothing and moisturizing properties that can calm an irritated scalp. Apply fresh aloe vera gel directly to your scalp, leave it on for 20-30 minutes, and then rinse thoroughly.

 - Apple Cider Vinegar Rinse: Apple cider vinegar helps balance the scalp's pH levels, remove product buildup, and reduce dandruff. Mix one part apple cider vinegar with two parts water, apply it to your scalp after shampooing, leave it on for a few minutes, and rinse well.

 - Tea Tree Oil: Tea tree oil has antimicrobial properties that can help prevent scalp infections and reduce dandruff. Add a few drops of tea tree oil to your shampoo or dilute it with a carrier oil and apply it directly to your scalp.

3. Avoid Over-Washing: Washing your hair too frequently can strip the scalp of its natural oils,

leading to dryness and irritation. Aim to wash your hair 2-3 times a week, depending on your hair type and scalp condition. When washing, use lukewarm water instead of hot water to prevent further drying.

4. Exfoliate the Scalp: Just like your skin, your scalp can benefit from exfoliation to remove dead skin cells and promote healthy hair growth. Use a gentle scalp scrub or a brush with soft bristles to exfoliate your scalp once a week.

Hair Care Routine

Choosing the right hair care products and establishing a consistent routine are essential for maintaining the health and appearance of your hair. Here's how to create a hair care routine that supports healthy hair:

1. Shampoos and Conditioners: Opt for sulfate-free shampoos and conditioners that are gentle on the hair and scalp. Sulfates can strip the hair of its natural oils, leading to dryness and damage. Look for products that are enriched with nourishing ingredients like keratin, argan oil, or shea butter to strengthen and hydrate your hair.

2. Oils and Serums: Incorporating hair oils and serums into your routine can help protect your hair from environmental damage, reduce frizz, and add shine. Popular options include argan oil, coconut oil, and jojoba oil. Apply a small amount to the ends of your hair after washing or as a leave-in treatment.

3. Avoid Heat Styling: Excessive heat styling can weaken hair, causing it to become brittle and

prone to breakage. When possible, allow your hair to air dry naturally. If you must use heat styling tools, always apply a heat protectant spray and use the lowest heat setting necessary.

4. Trimming: Regular trims every 6-8 weeks help remove split ends and prevent further damage. This keeps your hair looking healthy and encourages growth.

5. Avoid Tight Hairstyles: Wearing your hair in tight ponytails, buns, or braids can cause tension on the hair shaft, leading to breakage and hair loss over time. Opt for looser hairstyles that don't put stress on your hair follicles.

Protective Hairstyles

As we age, our hair may become more fragile, making it essential to adopt hairstyles that minimize damage and protect the hair. Protective hairstyles are particularly beneficial for reducing breakage and maintaining hair health. Here are some protective hairstyle options and practices:

1. Loose Buns and Braids: Loose buns, braids, and twists are gentle on the hair and help prevent tangling and breakage. These styles keep your hair secure without pulling on the roots, making them ideal for everyday wear.

2. Silk or Satin Scarves: Wrapping your hair in a silk or satin scarf before bed can protect it from friction and breakage. Unlike cotton, silk and satin reduce hair friction, helping to maintain moisture and prevent split ends. You can also use a silk or satin pillowcase for additional protection.

3. Low-Manipulation Styles: Low-manipulation styles, such as leaving your hair down or in a loose ponytail, require minimal styling and reduce the risk of hair damage. These styles allow your hair to rest and recover between more elaborate hairstyles.

4. Clip-In Extensions: If you want to add length or volume to your hair without damaging your natural strands, consider using clip-in extensions. These temporary extensions are easy to apply and remove, allowing you to switch up your hairstyle without the risk of damage.

DIY Hair Masks and Treatments

Homemade hair masks using natural ingredients can provide deep nourishment and hydration to your hair. These treatments are easy to make and offer a cost-effective way to improve the health and appearance of your hair. Here are some DIY hair mask recipes to try:

1. Avocado and Honey Mask

- Ingredients: 1 ripe avocado, 2 tablespoons honey, 1 tablespoon olive oil

- Instructions: Mash the avocado until smooth, then mix in the honey and olive oil. Apply the mask to damp hair, focusing on the ends. Leave it on for 20-30 minutes, then rinse thoroughly and shampoo as usual. This mask is rich in fatty acids and vitamins, making it ideal for dry, damaged hair.

2. Yogurt and Egg Mask

   - Ingredients: 1/2 cup plain yogurt, 1 egg, 1 tablespoon coconut oil

   - Instructions: Whisk the egg in a bowl, then add the yogurt and coconut oil. Mix until well combined. Apply the mask to your hair, covering it from roots to ends. Leave it on for 20-30 minutes, then rinse with cool water and shampoo. The protein in the egg strengthens hair, while the yogurt and coconut oil provide moisture and shine.

3. Banana and Olive Oil Mask

   - Ingredients: 1 ripe banana, 2 tablespoons olive oil, 1 tablespoon honey

   - Instructions: Blend the banana until smooth, then mix in the olive oil and honey.

Apply the mask to your hair, focusing on any areas that need extra moisture. Leave it on for 20-30 minutes, then rinse thoroughly and shampoo. This mask is great for smoothing frizz and adding shine.

4. Aloe Vera and Coconut Milk Mask

  - Ingredients: 1/4 cup aloe vera gel, 1/4 cup coconut milk, 1 tablespoon almond oil

  - Instructions: Mix the aloe vera gel, coconut milk, and almond oil in a bowl. Apply the mask to your hair and scalp, massaging it in gently. Leave it on for 20-30 minutes, then rinse thoroughly and shampoo. This mask soothes the scalp and deeply conditions the hair.

5. Oatmeal and Almond Oil Mask

   - Ingredients: 1/4 cup oatmeal (finely ground), 1/4 cup almond oil, 2 tablespoons honey

   - Instructions: Combine the ground oatmeal, almond oil, and honey in a bowl. Apply the mixture to damp hair, focusing on dry areas. Leave it on for 20-30 minutes, then rinse thoroughly and shampoo. This mask is especially beneficial for soothing an itchy scalp and moisturizing dry hair.

By incorporating these holistic hair care practices into your routine, you can maintain the health and vitality of your hair as you age. A healthy scalp, the right hair care products, protective hairstyles, and nourishing DIY treatments all work together to support your hair's natural beauty. Combined with a balanced diet rich in hair-friendly nutrients, these practices will help you achieve and maintain strong, vibrant, and healthy hair for years to come.

Personalizing Your Anti-Grey Hair Journey

Maintaining your hair color and health involves more than just following general advice. It's important to personalize your approach based on your individual needs, monitor your progress, and stay motivated throughout the process. This chapter provides guidance on how to tailor your diet and lifestyle to meet your specific needs, track your progress effectively, and stay inspired as you work toward your goals.

Identifying Your Nutritional Needs

Tailoring your diet to address specific hair concerns requires an understanding of your unique health history and lifestyle. Here's how to personalize your approach:

1. Assess Your Current Diet: Begin by evaluating your current eating habits. Take note of your daily intake of vitamins, minerals, and other nutrients that are important for hair health. Identify any gaps or deficiencies that may need to be addressed.

2. Consider Health Conditions: Certain health conditions, such as thyroid disorders, anemia, or hormonal imbalances, can affect hair color and health. If you have any existing health conditions, consult with a healthcare professional to determine how these might influence your hair and what specific dietary adjustments may be beneficial.

3. Evaluate Lifestyle Factors: Your lifestyle can also impact your hair health. Factors such as stress levels, sleep patterns, and physical

activity can all play a role. Consider how these factors might be affecting your hair and how you can adjust your diet and lifestyle to support better hair health.

4. Personalize Your Nutrient Intake: Based on your assessment, adjust your diet to include foods that address your specific needs. For example, if you're deficient in B vitamins, focus on incorporating more sources of these nutrients into your meals. If stress is a major factor, include foods rich in antioxidants and stress-reducing nutrients.

5. Consult a Nutritionist: If you're unsure about how to tailor your diet effectively, consider consulting a nutritionist or dietitian. They can provide personalized advice and help you

create a meal plan that meets your individual needs and goals.

Tracking Progress

Monitoring changes in your hair color and health is an essential part of your anti-grey hair journey. Here's how to track your progress effectively:

1. Keep a Hair Journal: Document your hair's condition regularly by keeping a journal. Record details such as changes in color, texture, and overall health. Note any new dietary changes or lifestyle adjustments you've made. This can help you identify patterns and assess the effectiveness of your approach.

2. Take Before-and-After Photos: Photograph your hair at regular intervals to visually track changes over time. This can provide a clear

comparison and help you see subtle improvements that may not be immediately noticeable.

3. Monitor Nutrient Levels: If you're making significant dietary changes, consider getting periodic blood tests to check your nutrient levels. This can help you determine if you're meeting your nutritional needs and make any necessary adjustments.

4. Evaluate Hair Health: Pay attention to how your hair feels and behaves. Notice if it's becoming stronger, shinier, or less prone to breakage. These indicators can provide valuable insights into the effectiveness of your dietary and lifestyle changes.

5. Consult a Healthcare Professional: If you experience significant changes in your hair

health or if you're unsure about your progress, consult a healthcare professional. They can offer additional guidance and help you address any underlying issues.

Staying Motivated

Maintaining commitment to your anti-grey hair diet and lifestyle changes can be challenging. Here are some tips for staying motivated and inspired throughout your journey:

1. Set Realistic Goals: Establish achievable goals for your hair health and color maintenance. Break these goals into smaller, manageable steps to make them feel more attainable. Celebrate your progress along the way to stay motivated.

2. Find Support: Connect with others who share similar goals or challenges. Joining support

groups, online forums, or social media communities focused on hair health can provide encouragement and inspiration.

3. Learn from Success Stories: Read about others who have successfully maintained or improved their hair color and health through diet and lifestyle changes. Their stories can offer motivation and practical tips that you can apply to your own journey.

4. Create a Routine: Develop a consistent routine for your hair care and dietary practices. Establishing habits makes it easier to stay on track and integrate these changes into your daily life.

5. Reward Yourself: Acknowledge and reward yourself for sticking to your plan and making positive changes. This could be through small

treats, self-care activities, or simply recognizing your achievements.

6. Stay Positive: Focus on the positive changes you're making and the benefits you're experiencing. A positive mindset can help you overcome challenges and stay committed to your goals.

By personalizing your anti-grey hair journey, tracking your progress, and staying motivated, you can effectively work towards maintaining your hair's color and health. Embrace this journey with patience and perseverance, and remember that every positive step you take contributes to achieving your desired results.

Conclusion

Embracing the Journey

As we age, it's natural for changes to occur, including the graying of our hair. This process, while a normal part of aging, doesn't mean we have to resign ourselves to feeling less vibrant or confident. By taking proactive steps to maintain our hair health through a balanced diet and holistic care practices, we can support our hair's natural beauty and vitality.

Embracing the journey of aging involves understanding and accepting these changes while actively working to enhance our overall well-being. It's about finding a balance between honoring our natural process and making choices that help us feel our best. Remember, the goal isn't just to maintain a youthful appearance but to cultivate a sense of confidence and self-love that radiates from within.

The Power of Consistency

The key to achieving long-term benefits from dietary and lifestyle changes lies in consistency. Incorporating hair-healthy nutrients into your diet, practicing good scalp care, and adopting supportive lifestyle habits are all steps that, when maintained regularly, can lead to noticeable improvements in hair health.

Consistency doesn't mean perfection; it's about making sustained efforts and adapting as needed. By sticking to your personalized plan and making these practices a regular part of your routine, you'll be more likely to see positive results over time. Celebrate the small victories and recognize the progress you're making along the way.

Final Thoughts

Aging gracefully is about more than just how we look; it's about how we feel and how we carry ourselves. As you continue your journey to maintain your hair's health and color, remember to stay motivated and confident. Your commitment to a healthy lifestyle and positive self-image is a testament to your strength and resilience.

Approach each day with a sense of pride in your ability to take charge of your well-being. Aging is a beautiful process, and with the right mindset and practices, you can continue to feel vibrant, confident, and empowered. Embrace every stage of life with grace and joy, knowing that you are making choices that enhance your health and beauty.

Appendices

Appendix A: Nutrient Reference Guide

This quick-reference chart provides a summary of key nutrients important for hair health, their food sources, and their roles in maintaining hair color and overall vitality.

Nutrient: B Vitamins

Food Sources: Eggs, leafy greens, whole grains, nuts, seeds

Role in Hair Health: Supports melanin production, strengthens hair strands, and aids in overall scalp health

Nutrient: Vitamin B12

Food Sources: Meat, dairy products, fortified cereals

Role in Hair Health: Essential for red blood cell production and overall hair health

Nutrient: Folic Acid

Food Sources: Leafy greens, legumes, citrus fruits

Role in Hair Health: Supports cell division and hair growth

Nutrient: Biotin

Food Sources: Eggs, nuts, seeds, sweet potatoes

Role in Hair Health: Promotes healthy hair growth and reduces hair loss

Nutrient: Copper

Food Sources: Shellfish, nuts, seeds, whole grains

Role in Hair Health: Contributes to melanin production and hair pigmentation

Nutrient: Iron

Food Sources: Red meat, beans, spinach, fortified cereals

Role in Hair Health: Essential for oxygen transport to hair follicles, reducing hair loss

Nutrient: Vitamin C

Food Sources: Citrus fruits, strawberries, bell peppers

Role in Hair Health: Acts as an antioxidant, aiding in the absorption of iron and combating oxidative stress

Nutrient: Vitamin E

Food Sources: Nuts, seeds, spinach, avocado

Role in Hair Health: Protects hair from oxidative damage and supports scalp health

Nutrient: Selenium

Food Sources: Brazil nuts, seafood, eggs, whole grains

Role in Hair Health: Acts as an antioxidant, protecting hair follicles from damage

Nutrient: Omega-3 Fatty Acids

Food Sources: Fatty fish, flaxseeds, walnuts

Role in Hair Health: Supports scalp health, reduces inflammation, and adds shine to hair

Nutrient: Protein

Food Sources: Meat, fish, dairy, legumes, nuts

Role in Hair Health: Essential for hair structure and strength

Nutrient: Tyrosine

Food Sources: Soy products, dairy, nuts, meats

Role in Hair Health: An amino acid important for melanin production

Appendix B: Recipe Ideas

Here are additional recipe ideas to help you explore more ways to incorporate anti-grey hair foods into your diet:

1. Spinach and Feta Stuffed Chicken Breasts

- Ingredients: Chicken breasts, spinach, feta cheese, garlic, olive oil

- Instructions: Sauté spinach and garlic in olive oil. Mix with crumbled feta cheese. Stuff chicken breasts with the mixture and bake until cooked through.

2. Quinoa and Black Bean Salad

- Ingredients: Quinoa, black beans, corn, cherry tomatoes, avocado, lime juice, cilantro

- Instructions: Cook quinoa according to package instructions. Mix with black beans, corn, chopped cherry tomatoes, and diced avocado. Toss with lime juice and cilantro.

3. Baked Salmon with Lemon and Dill

- Ingredients: Salmon fillets, lemon slices, fresh dill, olive oil, garlic

- Instructions: Place salmon fillets on a baking sheet. Top with lemon slices, dill, and a drizzle of olive oil. Bake until salmon is flaky.

4. Almond and Berry Smoothie

- Ingredients: Almond milk, mixed berries, almond butter, honey

- Instructions: Blend almond milk, mixed berries, a spoonful of almond butter, and a drizzle of honey until smooth.

5. Avocado and Tomato Toast

- Ingredients: Whole grain bread, ripe avocado, cherry tomatoes, olive oil, salt, pepper

- Instructions: Toast whole grain bread. Mash avocado and spread it over the toast. Top with sliced cherry tomatoes, a drizzle of olive oil, salt, and pepper.

Appendix C: Resources

For further reading and additional resources on hair health and aging, consider the following reputable websites and organizations:

Books:

- "The Science and Fine Art of Food and Nutrition" by Arnold Ehret

- "Hair Care Rehab: The Ultimate Hair Repair & Renewal Plan" by Audrey Davis-Sivasothy

Websites:

- American Academy of Dermatology (AAD): www.aad.org – Provides information on hair care and dermatological health.

- National Institutes of Health (NIH): www.nih.gov – Offers research and resources on various health topics, including nutrition and aging.

- Mayo Clinic: [www.mayoclinic.org](https://www.mayoclinic.

org) – Features articles and advice on hair health and dietary recommendations.

Organizations:

- American Hair Loss Association (AHLA): www.americanhairloss.org – Focuses on hair loss education and resources.

- International Society of Hair Restoration Surgery (ISHRS): www.ishrs.org – Provides information on hair restoration and health.

Disclaimer

The information provided in this book is for educational and informational purposes only and is not intended as medical advice. The contents of this book should not be used to diagnose, treat, or prevent any health condition or disease. Always consult with a qualified healthcare professional before making any significant changes to your diet, lifestyle, or health regimen, particularly if you have any pre-existing medical conditions, are pregnant, nursing, or taking medications.

The authors and publishers of this book are not responsible for any adverse effects or consequences resulting from the use of the suggestions, dietary practices, or any other information described in this book. Individual results may vary, and the effectiveness of dietary and lifestyle changes can differ based on a variety of factors, including genetics, overall health, and adherence to the recommended practices.

This book is not intended to replace professional medical advice, diagnosis, or treatment. If you have specific health concerns, please consult a healthcare provider to obtain personalized recommendations.

No part of this book may be reproduced, distributed, or transmitted in any form or by any means, including photocopying, recording, or other electronic or mechanical methods, without the prior written permission of the author, except in the case of brief quotations embodied in critical reviews and certain other noncommercial uses permitted by copyright law.

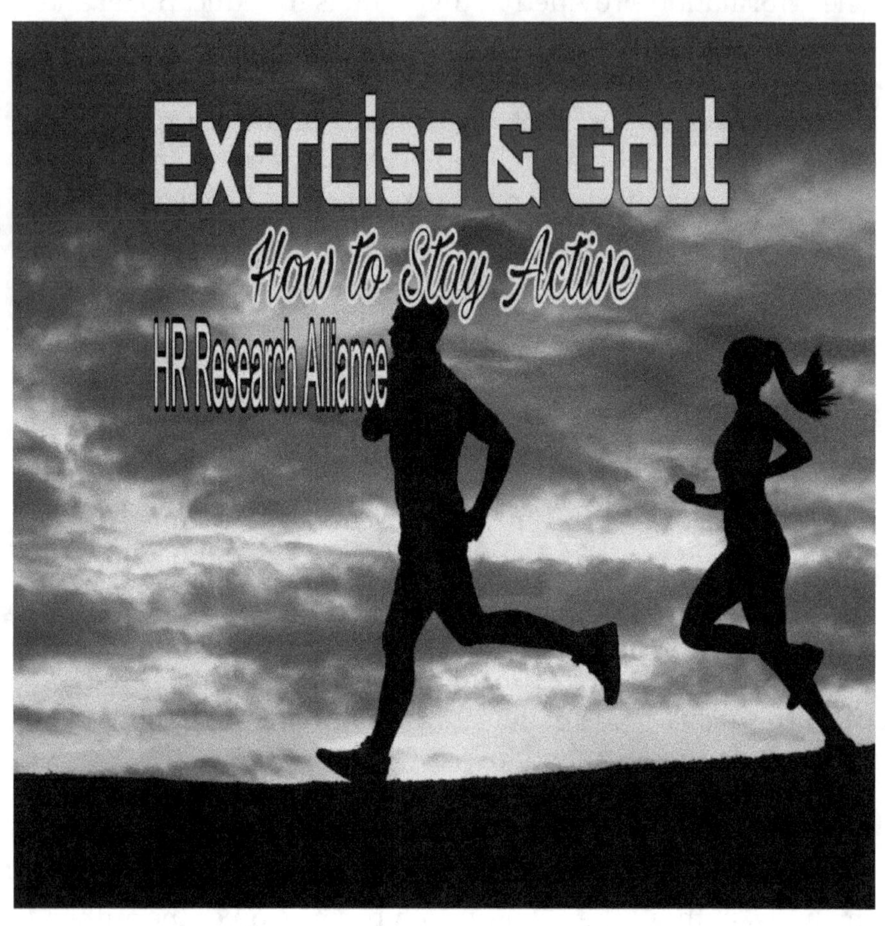

Search HR Research Alliance wherever Books, Audiobooks, eBooks are sold.